The Bath Bomb Rec_

Written by Erin Anderson

Disclaimer:

The information contained in this book is for general information purposes only.

While we endeavor to keep the information up to date and correct, we make no representations or warranties of any kind, express or implied, about the completeness, accuracy, reliability, suitability or availability with respect to the book or the information, products, services, or related graphics contained in the book for any purpose. Any reliance you place on such information is therefore strictly at your own risk.

None of the information in this this book is meant to be construed as medical advice. Essential oils are powerful compounds. Consult with a medical professional prior to making changes that could impact your health.

Contents

Bath Bomb Basics

Bath bombs are compact little balls that bubble and fizz when they're tossed into a tub full of water. As they bubble, they release the contents of the bath bomb into the tub, filling it with the vegetable oils, butters, salts and essential oils contained inside.

They look like they're difficult to make, but once you get the hang of it, bath bombs are actually fairly easy to put together. That doesn't stop manufacturers from charging a premium for them, as they can cost a small fortune in the store, with some companies charging as much as $10 to $15 per bath bomb. When you make them at home, you can get the cost down to a buck or two per bath bomb.

There are only 6 ingredients that go into making a basic bath bomb:

- **Baking soda.**
- **Citric acid.**
- **Corn starch.**
- **Epsom salts.**
- **Vegetable oil.**
- **Water or witch hazel.**

Of those 6 ingredients, the 2 key ingredients are the baking soda and the citric acid because they're the ingredients that make the magic happen. Combine them when they're dry and nothing happens. Add water to the equation and a chemical reaction occurs that creates carbon dioxide. The effect you get when you throw a bath bomb in the tub is similar to that of carbonation in a soda, as the carbon dioxide bubbles pour out of the bath bomb and into the water.

The corn starch is added to provide buoyancy, as most people prefer their bath bombs to float at the top of the tub. When the corn starch is left out, a bath bomb will still create bubbles; it'll just do so from the bottom of the tub.

Epsom salts are added to provide volume and because they're good for the skin and for the body. A bath with Epsom salts in it is relaxing and can help relieve stress. Other natural salts like Himalayan pink sea salt can be substituted for the Epsom salt to good effect.

Vegetable oils are used as carrier oils to disperse the essential oils and other bath bomb ingredients into the tub. These carrier oils carry essential oils deep within the skin, where they can be absorbed into the blood stream and carried throughout the body. Certain butters can also be added to bath bombs to ensure they moisturize the skin and leave it feeling supple and smooth.

The last ingredient required to make bath bombs is either water or witch hazel. This ingredient is added to the bath bomb mixture to make sure it's damp enough to where it can be pressed into the mold and will retain its shape until it's had a chance to dry. When adding water or witch hazel to a recipe, it's important to only add a little bit at a time or you could set off the reaction between the baking soda and the citric acid. If this happens and you start to see bubbles, you can usually stop the reaction by quickly stirring the area that's bubbling.

All other ingredients are optional, and are added to create a certain effect. Dyes, clays and other colorants can be added to fill the tub with color; essential oils and fragrance oils can be added for scent; and dried herbs and flowers can be added as garnish. We'll discuss a number of these ingredients as we use them in the recipes.

Safety Precaution: The Power of Essential Oils

You'll notice that a large number of the recipes in this book call for essential oils. Essential oils are the powerful aromatic essence of plants and are used to add fragrance to the bath bombs, along with a number of other benefits. While fragrance oils are available and are generally cheaper than essential oils, I prefer using essential oils whenever possible because they're entirely natural and don't contain potentially-dangerous synthetic chemicals. Some of the recipes in this book do call for use of fragrance oils, but that's only when an acceptable essential oil or oil blend isn't available to create the desired fragrance.

Just because essential oils are natural doesn't mean they aren't powerful. It can take tens of thousands of plants to make an ounce or two of essential oil, so you'd better believe this concentrated essence is powerful stuff. Use the right oil at the right time and it can provide therapeutic benefits. Using the wrong oil can result in skin irritation, inflammation and allergic reactions.

Consult with your physician before beginning use of essential oils. This is especially-important if you take prescription medications, since essential oils can dull or enhance the effects of certain drugs. It's also important to discuss essential oils with your doctor if you have underlying health conditions, are pregnant or you want to use them on younger children.

Use essential oils at your own risk. The information covered in future chapters is not a complete list of the benefits and dangers of essential oils by any means. Entire books have been written on them and this book only covers the oils used in recipes to the degree in which they're to be used.

It's up to you to research new oils and decide whether they're a good fit. When and if you do decide to add a new oil to your bath bombs, always dilute the new oil and test it on a small patch of skin to see if irritation occurs. If it does, discontinue use of that oil immediately.

Safety Precaution: Slip Hazard

There aren't too many things more relaxing than slipping into a tub into which a bath bomb has been released. What isn't so relaxing is actually slipping as you get in or out of the tub. One inherent danger associated with filling a tub full of oils and melted butters is the increased risk of taking a tumble while climbing in and out of the tub.

The smooth surfaces of the tub will become extremely slippery once the oils and butters come in contact with them, so it's important to be careful to make sure you don't fall. Non-slip bath mats will help, but even then things can get a bit slippery. Be careful and make sure your movements are slow and calculated. It's best to ease yourself in and out of the tub.

You don't want bath time to turn into a trip to the emergency room!

The Beginner's Bath Bomb

Let's start off with the basics. This recipe is the basis for the rest of the recipes in the book and you aren't going to see much deviation from this recipe as far as the key ingredients are concerned. The good news is once you're able to make this bath bomb, the rest should be a breeze because they aren't that much different.

This recipe uses sweet almond oil as the carrier oil. It's one of the most-used oils in bath bombs because it's easily absorbed and doesn't leave you feeling greasy when you get out of the tub. It smells slightly nutty and has the faintest fragrance of the almonds it's derived from, but once you add essential oils to it, you usually can't smell it at all.

Ingredients:

2 cups baking soda
1 cup citric acid
¼ cup Epsom salt
¼ cup corn starch
1 tablespoon sweet almond oil
Water or witch hazel

Directions:

1. Combine the baking soda, citric acid, Epsom salt and corn starch. Make sure they're thoroughly blended.
2. Add the sweet almond oil to the dry ingredients and stir it in.

3. Add water or witch hazel to a spray bottle and use it to lightly mist the bath bomb mixture. Use your hands to knead the liquid in until the mixture is slightly damp and is able to hold its form when you squeeze a ball of it in your hand.

4. Press the mixture into your bath bomb molds. Pack it as tightly as possible

5. Remove the bath bombs from the molds and place them in a cool, dry place for a day or two until they've had time to finish drying.

6. Store them in an airtight container in a cool, dry place.

The Oatmeal Bath Bomb

Here's another base recipe you can use when making bath bombs. This recipe substitutes half of the corn starch for ground oatmeal. The result is a milky bath that leaves your skin feeling silky smooth.

The essential oils you add are left up to you with this recipe. If you're new to the world of essential oils, try adding 10 drops of lavender oil.

Ingredients:

2 cups baking soda
1 cup citric acid
¼ cup Epsom salt
2 tablespoons corn starch
2 tablespoons ground oatmeal
1 tablespoon sweet almond oil
Water or witch hazel

Directions:

1. Combine the baking soda, citric acid, Epsom salt, ground oatmeal and corn starch. Make sure they're thoroughly blended.
2. Add the sweet almond oil to the dry ingredients and stir it in.
3. Add water or witch hazel to a spray bottle and use it to lightly mist the bath bomb mixture. Use your hands to knead the liquid in until the

mixture is slightly damp and is able to hold its form when you squeeze a ball of it in your hand.

4. Press the mixture into your bath bomb molds. Pack it as tightly as possible

5. Remove the bath bombs from the molds and place them in a cool, dry place for a day or two until they've had time to finish drying.

6. Store them in an airtight container in a cool, dry place.

Lavender Fields

This is the first recipe that calls for an essential oil, and it's one you're going to want to familiarize yourself with. Lavender essential oil is one of the milder essential oils and can be used by most people. While this recipe calls for just lavender oil, it can be blended with most other oils to good effect. Lavender oil by itself is good, but when it's blended with other oils, it enhances their fragrance and make them even better.

There's good reason lavender essential oil is one of the most popular essential oils around. It's a healing oil that can be used to help heal minor cuts, scrapes, scratches, burns, sunburns and insect bites. Lavender oil is anti-inflammatory and can help alleviate a number of skin conditions. It's got a soothing floral fragrance and can be used to help you wind down after a long day.

The dried lavender flowers in this recipe are primarily there for aesthetic value. You can leave them out and still realize the benefits of lavender essential oil.

Ingredients:

2 cups baking soda
1 cup citric acid
¼ cup Epsom salt
¼ cup corn starch
1 tablespoon sweet almond oil
15 drops lavender essential oil
Water or witch hazel
Dried lavender flowers

Optional: Natural purple clay

Directions:

1. Combine the baking soda, citric acid, Epsom salt and corn starch. Make sure they're thoroughly blended.
2. Combine the lavender essential oil and almond oil and stir it into the dry ingredients.
3. If you're planning on coloring the bath bombs, add the natural purple clay at this time and stir it in. Only use as much as it takes to achieve the desired color.
4. Add water or witch hazel to a spray bottle and use it to lightly mist the bath bomb mixture. Use your hands to knead the liquid in until the mixture is slightly damp and is able to hold its form when you squeeze a ball of it in your hand.
5. Crumble the lavender flowers and add a small amount of flowers to the bottom of each of the molds. Alternatively, you can add them to the bath bomb mixture and stir them in before pressing the mixture into the molds.
6. Press the mixture into your bath bomb molds. Pack the molds as tightly as possible
7. Remove the bath bombs from the molds and place them in a cool, dry place for a day or two until they've had time to finish drying.
8. Store them in an airtight container in a cool, dry place.

Cinnamon Oatmeal Bombs

This recipe builds on the previous one by adding cinnamon to the mix. I've seen recipes that call for cinnamon essential oil instead of the cinnamon tea used in this recipe, but I prefer the light smell of cinnamon you get from the tea, as opposed to the strong fragrance of the essential oil. I've also added some ground cinnamon to this recipe to further up the amount of cinnamon used and to give the bath bomb a marbled texture.

Cinnamon is good for the skin and can be used to restore elasticity and shine to dry, damaged skin. It can also be used to help clear up stubborn cases of acne. It improves blood flow into the small capillaries of the skin and may help remove fine wrinkles by adding a bit of volume to the skin.

All you need now is some powdered milk and sugar and you'll be bathing in your breakfast!

Ingredients:

2 cups baking soda
1 cup citric acid
¼ cup Epsom salt
2 tablespoons corn starch
2 tablespoons ground oatmeal
2 tablespoons strong cinnamon tea
1 tablespoon ground cinnamon
1 tablespoon sweet almond oil
Water or witch hazel

Directions:

1. Combine the baking soda, citric acid, Epsom salt, ground oatmeal and corn starch. Make sure they're thoroughly blended.
2. Brew some strong cinnamon tea. Add the sweet almond oil and cinnamon tea to the dry ingredients and stir them in.
3. Add water or witch hazel to a spray bottle and use it to lightly mist the bath bomb mixture. Use your hands to knead the liquid in until the mixture is slightly damp and is able to hold its form when you squeeze a ball of it in your hand.
4. Press the mixture into your bath bomb molds. Layer the ground cinnamon into the molds for a marbled effect. Pack the molds as tightly as possible
5. Remove the bath bombs from the molds and place them in a cool, dry place for a day or two until they've had time to finish drying.
6. Store them in an airtight container in a cool, dry place.

Cocoa Butter Moisturizing Bombs

This bath bomb uses cocoa butter and Shea butter to create a bath bomb that moisturizes the skin. Cocoa butter is made up of fats taken from cocoa beans and has the light fragrance of chocolate. Shea butter is a solid butter that can be used to help firm up your bath bombs while adding moisturizing properties.

I prefer to use this bath bomb in its unscented form, but I have been known to roll it in cacao powder after pulling it out of the mold. Another option is to layer the cacao powder into the mold with the bath bomb mixture to create a marbled effect. The cacao powder isn't just there for looks. It contains a number of minerals that are beneficial to the skin and the caffeine in the cacao powder may help tighten and condition the skin.

This recipe calls for coconut oil, which is an inexpensive oil that's a solid at cooler temperatures, but will become liquid when temperatures start to climb. It conditions the skin and has emollient properties, so it can be used to disperse other ingredients into the water.

Ingredients:

2 cups baking soda
1 cup citric acid
¼ cup Epsom salt
¼ cup corn starch
1 tablespoon cacao powder
1 tablespoon coconut oil
Water or witch hazel

Directions:

1. Combine the baking soda, citric acid, Epsom salt and corn starch. Make sure they're thoroughly blended.
2. Melt the coconut oil, if it isn't already melted. Add the coconut oil to the dry ingredients and stir it in.
3. Add water or witch hazel to a spray bottle and use it to lightly mist the bath bomb mixture. Use your hands to knead the liquid in until the mixture is slightly damp and is able to hold its form when you squeeze a ball of it in your hand.
4. Press the mixture into your bath bomb molds. Layer the cacao powder in thin layers in the molds. Pack the molds as tightly as possible
5. Remove the bath bombs from the molds and place them in a cool, dry place for a day or two until they've had time to finish drying.
6. Store them in an airtight container in a cool, dry place.

Thrilla in Vanilla

Sorry about the cheesy name, but I couldn't think of anything else that rhymed with vanilla that was a good fit for this bath bomb. If you love vanilla, you're going to love the way this bath bomb fills the bathroom with the fragrance of vanilla.

This recipe calls for vanilla absolute, since there is no pure form of vanilla essential oil. Don't be fooled by the companies online claiming to sell pure vanilla essential oil. Vanilla oil isn't steam-distilled or cold-pressed from the beans, so it isn't pure. Vanilla absolute is extracted from the beans of the vanilla plant using solvents or carbon dioxide and is as close as you're going to get to the real thing. Luckily, it has the strong fragrance of vanilla and works well in bath products, granted you only use a tiny amount.

The sugar is there for looks and won't do much in the tub because such a small amount is used. It does add a light, sweet fragrance to the bath bombs. Try adding other essential oils to this bath bomb to further enhance the fragrance. Lavender oil works well, as do a number of citrus oils.

Ingredients:

2 cups baking soda
1 cup citric acid
¼ cup Epsom salt
¼ cup corn starch
1 tablespoon extra-virgin coconut oil
A few drops of vanilla absolute

1 teaspoon white rock crystal sugar
Water or witch hazel

Directions:

1. Combine the baking soda, citric acid, Epsom salt and corn starch. Make sure they're thoroughly blended.
2. Gently melt the coconut oil if it's solid. Add the vanilla absolute to the coconut oil and stir it in.
3. Add water or witch hazel to a spray bottle and use it to lightly mist the bath bomb mixture. Use your hands to knead the liquid in until the mixture is slightly damp and is able to hold its form when you squeeze a ball of it in your hand.
4. Add several sugar crystals to each of the molds.
5. Press the mixture into your bath bomb molds. Pack the molds as tightly as possible
6. Remove the bath bombs from the molds and place them in a cool, dry place for a day or two until they've had time to finish drying.
7. Store them in an airtight container in a cool, dry place.

Vanilla Cocoa Cream

This is one of the more luxurious bath bombs, as you're left with a tub full of cocoa butter and coconut oil to soak in once the bomb has done its thing. Your skin will be moisturized while the room fills with the fragrance of chocolate and vanilla.

If you'd like a completely natural option that smells similar to, but not exactly the same as, vanilla then balsam peru essential oil can be used.

Ingredients:

2 cups baking soda
1 cup citric acid
¼ cup Epsom salt
¼ cup corn starch
1 tablespoon cocoa powder
1 tablespoon extra-virgin coconut oil
1 tablespoon cocoa butter
A few drops of vanilla absolute
Water or witch hazel

Directions:

1. Combine the baking soda, citric acid, cocoa powder, Epsom salt and corn starch. Make sure they're thoroughly blended.
2. Gently melt the coconut oil and cocoa butter. Add the vanilla absolute to the oil and butter mixture and stir it in.

3. Add water or witch hazel to a spray bottle and use it to lightly mist the bath bomb mixture. Use your hands to knead the liquid in until the mixture is slightly damp and is able to hold its form when you squeeze a ball of it in your hand.
4. Press the mixture into your bath bomb molds. Pack the molds as tightly as possible
5. Remove the bath bombs from the molds and place them in a cool, dry place for a day or two until they've had time to finish drying.
6. Store them in an airtight container in a cool, dry place.

Orange Cream

The orange cream bath bomb takes two different citrus oils and blends them into a bath bomb that has powdered soy milk added to it to create a silky and luxurious bath time experience that smells surprisingly similar to that of an orange cream soda. While I'm not a huge fan of soy milk as far as using it as a beverage goes, it does have its benefits as an ingredient in bath products, as it moisturizes the skin and will leave your body feeling silky smooth.

Citrus essential oils have astringent properties that will tighten up loose skin and will help clear up oily skin. They're uplifting and energizing and will leave you and your tub smelling citrus fresh. Be aware that citrus oils can be phototoxic by nature. Don't use this bath bomb when you plan on being exposed to the sun within the next 24 hours.

Ingredients:

2 cups baking soda
1 cup citric acid
¼ cup Epsom salt
¼ cup corn starch
2 tablespoons powdered soy milk
1 tablespoon sweet almond oil
5 drops orange essential oil
5 drops bergamot essential oil
Water or witch hazel
OPTIONAL: Natural orange clay, for coloring

Directions:

1. Combine the baking soda, citric acid, Epsom salt, powdered soy milk and corn starch. Make sure they're thoroughly blended. Add the orange clay at this time and blend it in, if you plan on coloring the bath bomb.

2. Add the essential oils to the sweet almond oil and stir them in.

3. Add water or witch hazel to a spray bottle and use it to lightly mist the bath bomb mixture. Use your hands to knead the liquid in until the mixture is slightly damp and is able to hold its form when you squeeze a ball of it in your hand.

4. Press the mixture into your bath bomb molds. Pack the molds as tightly as possible

5. Remove the bath bombs from the molds and place them in a cool, dry place for a day or two until they've had time to finish drying.

6. Store them in an airtight container in a cool, dry place.

Creamy Avocado

The fresh avocado and the avocado oil used in this recipe make the bathwater feel silky smooth and your skin will feel the same way when you leave the tub. Since there isn't much by way of fragrance when it comes to avocado or avocado oil, I've added lemongrass oil to the recipe for a refreshing fragrance that leaves you feeling rejuvenated and energized.

Ingredients:

2 cups baking soda
1 cup citric acid
¼ cup Epsom salt
¼ cup corn starch
2 tablespoons mashed avocado
1 tablespoon avocado oil
10 drops lemongrass oil
Water or witch hazel
OPTIONAL: Natural green clay, for coloring

Directions:

1. Combine the baking soda, citric acid, Epsom salt, and corn starch. Make sure they're thoroughly blended. Add the green clay at this time and blend it in, if you plan on coloring the bath bomb.

2. Combine the mashed avocado, avocado oil and lemongrass oil and work it into the dry ingredients. Remove any lumps that form.
3. Add water or witch hazel to a spray bottle and use it to lightly mist the bath bomb mixture. Use your hands to knead the liquid in until the mixture is slightly damp and is able to hold its form when you squeeze a ball of it in your hand.
4. Press the mixture into your bath bomb molds. Pack the molds as tightly as possible
5. Remove the bath bombs from the molds and place them in a cool, dry place for a day or two until they've had time to finish drying.
6. Store them in an airtight container in a cool, dry place.

The Deep Thinker

If you're the type of person who uses bath time as a time to relax and think back through the issues that presented themselves the previous day, this bath bomb is a great choice. It uses three different essential oils to create a soothing fragrance that's relaxing and will help you navigate through stressful times.

The combination of lavender, sandalwood and rose geranium essential oils in this bath bomb is soothing to the mind, the body and the soul. They're also pretty good for your skin, so you'll leave the bath feeling great.

Ingredients:

2 cups baking soda
1 cup citric acid
¼ cup Epsom salt
¼ cup corn starch
1 tablespoon cocoa butter
10 drops lavender essential oil
5 drops sandalwood essential oil
5 drops rose geranium essential oil
Water or witch hazel

Directions:

1. Combine the baking soda, citric acid, Epsom salt and corn starch. Make sure they're thoroughly blended.

2. Melt the cocoa butter. Stir in the essential oils. Add the wet ingredients to the dry ingredients and mix them in.

3. Add water or witch hazel to a spray bottle and use it to lightly mist the bath bomb mixture. Use your hands to knead the liquid in until the mixture is slightly damp and is able to hold its form when you squeeze a ball of it in your hand.

4. Press the mixture into your bath bomb molds. Pack the molds as tightly as possible

5. Remove the bath bombs from the molds and place them in a cool, dry place for a day or two until they've had time to finish drying.

6. Store them in an airtight container in a cool, dry place.

Baby Soft Skin

If you're looking for silky, smooth skin that's as soft as a baby's bottom, you've just found your new favorite bath bomb. The aloe vera butter, cocoa butter and avocado butter combine to moisturize the skin. The essential oil blend added to this bath bomb also helps moisturize the skin and should help rejuvenate dry, damaged skin that's worn from the effects of time and weather.

Try adding a tablespoon of ground oatmeal to this recipe to further enhance the skin softening properties.

Ingredients:

2 cups baking soda
1 cup citric acid
¼ cup Epsom salt
¼ cup corn starch
1 tablespoon cocoa butter
1 teaspoon aloe vera butter
1 teaspoon avocado butter
10 drops lavender essential oil
Water or witch hazel

Directions:

1. Combine the baking soda, citric acid, Epsom salt and corn starch. Make sure they're thoroughly blended.
2. Gently melt the butters. Add the lavender essential oil and stir it in.

3. Add water or witch hazel to a spray bottle and use it to lightly mist the bath bomb mixture. Use your hands to knead the liquid in until the mixture is slightly damp and is able to hold its form when you squeeze a ball of it in your hand.

4. Press the mixture into your bath bomb molds. Pack the molds as tightly as possible

5. Remove the bath bombs from the molds and place them in a cool, dry place for a day or two until they've had time to finish drying.

6. Store them in an airtight container in a cool, dry place.

Mature Skin Care

Sometimes your skin just needs pampering, especially for those amongst us who are approaching our golden years. The carrot seed oil in this recipe stimulates circulation and helps tone the skin, which may tighten up wrinkles. Some people swear by the anti-aging properties of this oil.

This bath bomb has a rich, earthy fragrance that you'll either love or hate. When buying carrot seed oil for the first time, only buy a small vial because it's a fragrance that not everyone is enamored with.

Ingredients:

2 cups baking soda
1 cup citric acid
¼ cup Epsom salt
¼ cup corn starch
1 tablespoon sweet almond oil
10 to 15 drops of carrot seed oil
Water or witch hazel

Directions:

1. Combine the baking soda, citric acid, Epsom salt and corn starch. Make sure they're thoroughly blended.
2. Combine the carrot seed oil and sweet almond oil and stir them together. Stir the wet ingredients and dry ingredients together.

3. Add water or witch hazel to a spray bottle and use it to lightly mist the bath bomb mixture. Use your hands to knead the liquid in until the mixture is slightly damp and is able to hold its form when you squeeze a ball of it in your hand.

4. Press the mixture into your bath bomb molds. Pack the molds as tightly as possible

5. Remove the bath bombs from the molds and place them in a cool, dry place for a day or two until they've had time to finish drying.

6. Store them in an airtight container in a cool, dry place.

The Fountain of Youth

This bath bomb features a blend of essential oils that nourish and protect the skin. A soak in the tub with this bath bomb should help tone the skin and you'll leave the tub feeling youthful and radiant.

Ingredients:

2 cups baking soda
1 cup citric acid
¼ cup Epsom salt
¼ cup corn starch
1 tablespoon sweet almond oil
5 drops Frankincense essential oil
5 drops myrhh essential oil
10 drops lavender essential oil
Water or witch hazel

Directions:

1. Combine the baking soda, citric acid, Epsom salt and corn starch. Make sure they're thoroughly blended.
2. Add the essential oils to the sweet almond oil and stir them in.
3. Add water or witch hazel to a spray bottle and use it to lightly mist the bath bomb mixture. Use your hands to knead the liquid in until the mixture is slightly damp and is able to hold its form when you squeeze a ball of it in your hand.

4. Press the mixture into your bath bomb molds. Pack the molds as tightly as possible

5. Remove the bath bombs from the molds and place them in a cool, dry place for a day or two until they've had time to finish drying.

6. Store them in an airtight container in a cool, dry place.

Black Licorice

I feel like a kid in a candy shop when I use this bath bomb, which uses star anise oil to create the fragrance of black licorice. Anise oil has a sedative effect, so it's best when used at the end of the day when you're trying to wind down.

As far as skin care goes, the combination of star anise oil and Shea butter in this recipe should leave your skin feeling soft and supple. It should also help moisturize the skin and has regenerative properties.

Ingredients:

2 cups baking soda
1 cup citric acid
¼ cup Epsom salt
¼ cup corn starch
1 tablespoon Shea butter
10 drops star anise essential oil
Dried whole star anise pods
Water or witch hazel

Directions:

1. Combine the baking soda, citric acid, Epsom salt and corn starch. Make sure they're thoroughly blended.
2. Gently melt the Shea butter. Add the star anise oil to the melted butter and stir it in.

3. Add water or witch hazel to a spray bottle and use it to lightly mist the bath bomb mixture. Use your hands to knead the liquid in until the mixture is slightly damp and is able to hold its form when you squeeze a ball of it in your hand.
4. Add one star anise to the bottom of each bath bomb mold. Press the mixture into your bath bomb molds. Pack the molds as tightly as possible
5. Remove the bath bombs from the molds and place them in a cool, dry place for a day or two until they've had time to finish drying.
6. Store them in an airtight container in a cool, dry place.

Minty Fresh

This easy-to-make bath bomb calls for peppermint essential oil, which is one of the more powerful essential oils that can be used in bath bombs. It smells similar to a candy cane, only stronger and with a more piercing fragrance. Peppermint oil can be used to ease congestion, relieve minor aches and pains and it's a cooling oil that might help reduce minor fevers.

Don't use too much peppermint oil in your bath bombs. This oil is one of the stronger oils and not everyone can tolerate it well.

Ingredients:

2 cups baking soda
1 cup citric acid
¼ cup Epsom salt
¼ cup corn starch
1 tablespoon extra-virgin coconut oil
10 drops peppermint essential oil
Water or witch hazel
Mint sprigs

Directions:

1. Combine the baking soda, citric acid, Epsom salt and corn starch. Make sure they're thoroughly blended.
2. Gently melt the coconut oil, if it's solid. Add the peppermint essential oil and stir it in.

3. Add water or witch hazel to a spray bottle and use it to lightly mist the bath bomb mixture. Use your hands to knead the liquid in until the mixture is slightly damp and is able to hold its form when you squeeze a ball of it in your hand.

4. Add a sprig of mint to the bottom of each of your molds.

5. Press the mixture into your bath bomb molds. Pack the molds as tightly as possible

6. Remove the bath bombs from the molds and place them in a cool, dry place for a day or two until they've had time to finish drying.

7. Store them in an airtight container in a cool, dry place.

Cold and Flu Relief

There are a number of essential oils that contain compounds that are decongestant and antiviral and antibacterial by nature. This recipe uses Roman chamomile, eucalyptus and peppermint essential oils to create a powerful oil blend that can help break up congestion and may ease the effects of the cold or the flu.

A short soak in the tub's all that's required when this bath bomb is in use. It's definitely on the strong side.

Ingredients:

2 cups baking soda
1 cup citric acid
¼ cup Epsom salt
¼ cup corn starch
1 tablespoon sweet almond oil
5 drops Roman chamomile essential oil
5 drops eucalyptus essential oil
5 drops peppermint essential oil
Water or witch hazel

Directions:

1. Combine the baking soda, citric acid, Epsom salt and corn starch. Make sure they're thoroughly blended.
2. Add the essential oils to the sweet almond oil and stir them in.

3. Add water or witch hazel to a spray bottle and use it to lightly mist the bath bomb mixture. Use your hands to knead the liquid in until the mixture is slightly damp and is able to hold its form when you squeeze a ball of it in your hand.

4. Press the mixture into your bath bomb molds. Pack the molds as tightly as possible

5. Remove the bath bombs from the molds and place them in a cool, dry place for a day or two until they've had time to finish drying.

6. Store them in an airtight container in a cool, dry place.

Breathe Easy

When you're feeling down in the dumps and a respiratory condition is causing problems breathing, a soak with this bath bomb might help you breathe easier. It's intended for use with minor respiratory conditions and should never be used in lieu of medical care for more serious ailments.

This one's a strong one and there's the potential for skin irritation, so a short soak is all that's recommended. Make sure your skin can tolerate these oils prior to using this bath bomb.

Ingredients:

2 cups baking soda
1 cup citric acid
¼ cup Epsom salt
¼ cup corn starch
1 tablespoon extra-virgin coconut oil
5 drops bay laurel essential oil
5 drops eucalyptus essential oil
Water or witch hazel

Directions:

1. Combine the baking soda, citric acid, Epsom salt and corn starch. Make sure they're thoroughly blended.
2. Gently melt the coconut oil if it's solid. Add the essential oils to the coconut oil and stir them in.

3. Add water or witch hazel to a spray bottle and use it to lightly mist the bath bomb mixture. Use your hands to knead the liquid in until the mixture is slightly damp and is able to hold its form when you squeeze a ball of it in your hand.

4. Press the mixture into your bath bomb molds. Pack the molds as tightly as possible

5. Remove the bath bombs from the molds and place them in a cool, dry place for a day or two until they've had time to finish drying.

6. Store them in an airtight container in a cool, dry place.

Citrus Surprise

Citrus essential oils are astringent oils that help tighten and tone the skin. They're antibacterial and antimicrobial by natural, so they can be used to help clear up infections. The fresh fragrance of this oil blend is uplifting and will leave you feeling refreshed and ready to take on anything life can throw your way.

Ingredients:

2 cups baking soda
1 cup citric acid
¼ cup Epsom salt
¼ cup corn starch
1 tablespoon coconut oil
5 drops mandarin essential oil
5 drops bergamot essential oil
5 drops lemon essential oil
Water or witch hazel

Directions:

1. Combine the baking soda, citric acid, Epsom salt and corn starch. Make sure they're thoroughly blended.
2. Gently melt the coconut oil if it's solid. Add the essential oils to the coconut oil and stir it in.
3. Add water or witch hazel to a spray bottle and use it to lightly mist the bath bomb mixture. Use your hands to knead the liquid in until the

mixture is slightly damp and is able to hold its form when you squeeze a ball of it in your hand.

4. Press the mixture into your bath bomb molds. Pack the molds as tightly as possible

5. Remove the bath bombs from the molds and place them in a cool, dry place for a day or two until they've had time to finish drying.

6. Store them in an airtight container in a cool, dry place.

Grandma's Kitchen

I've been using this recipe for a while, but struggled to come up with a name for it for this book. I finally settled on grandma's kitchen because when I lay back in the tub and close my eyes and breathe deeply, the spicy aroma reminds me of the way my grandma's kitchen used to smell around the holidays.

This recipe calls for black pepper essential oil, which is extracted from the unripe fruit of the Piper nigrum plant. When applied topically, black pepper oil is a warming oil that improves circulation and can be used to relieve muscle and joint pain. The fragrance is spicy and warm and is uplifting and stimulant. When combined with lemon essential oil, it's an effective blend to use when you have a long day ahead of you and you want to start it off feeling like you're ready to conquer the world.

Black pepper oil can cause irritation to those with sensitive skin, so always dilute it and test it before using it in your bath products.

Ingredients:

2 cups baking soda
1 cup citric acid
¼ cup Epsom salt
¼ cup corn starch
1 tablespoon coconut oil
5 drops black pepper oil
10 drops lemon essential oil
Water or witch hazel

Directions:

1. Combine the baking soda, citric acid, Epsom salt and corn starch. Make sure they're thoroughly blended.
2. Gently melt the coconut oil if it's solid. Add the essential oils to the coconut oil and stir them in.
3. Add water or witch hazel to a spray bottle and use it to lightly mist the bath bomb mixture. Use your hands to knead the liquid in until the mixture is slightly-damp and is able to hold its form when you squeeze a ball of it in your hand.
4. Press the mixture into your bath bomb molds. Pack the molds as tightly as possible
5. Remove the bath bombs from the molds and place them in a cool, dry place for a day or two until they've had time to finish drying.
6. Store them in an airtight container in a cool, dry place.

Ocean Breeze

I usually prefer essential oils to fragrance oils because of their many therapeutic benefits, but one smell that's tough to mimic using essential oils is the smell of a fresh ocean breeze. This recipe calls for an ocean breeze or ocean rain fragrance oil. There are a number of them on the market, so you'll have to experiment a bit to find one you like.

Ingredients:

2 cups baking soda
1 cup citric acid
¼ cup Epsom salt
¼ cup corn starch
1 teaspoon sea salt
1 tablespoon sweet almond oil
10 drops of ocean breeze or ocean rain fragrance oil
Water or witch hazel

Directions:

1. Combine the baking soda, citric acid, Epsom salt, sea salt and corn starch. Make sure they're thoroughly blended.
2. Add the fragrance oil to the sweet almond oil and stir it in.
3. Add water or witch hazel to a spray bottle and use it to lightly mist the bath bomb mixture. Use your hands to knead the liquid in until the

mixture is slightly damp and is able to hold its form when you squeeze a ball of it in your hand.

4. Press the mixture into your bath bomb molds. Pack the molds as tightly as possible

5. Remove the bath bombs from the molds and place them in a cool, dry place for a day or two until they've had time to finish drying.

6. Store them in an airtight container in a cool, dry place.

Passion Bath Bombs

All three of the essential oils used in these bath bombs are said to have aphrodisiac properties. I'm not sure how well they'll work for that purpose, but one thing's for sure...They smell great and your significant other will have a tough time keeping his hands off you after a bath with one of these bath bombs in it.

Ingredients:

2 cups baking soda
1 cup citric acid
¼ cup Epsom salt
2 tablespoons corn starch
1 tablespoon sweet almond oil
5 drops sandalwood essential oil
5 drops Mandarin essential oil
5 drops jasmine essential oil
Water or witch hazel

Directions:

1. Combine the baking soda, citric acid, Epsom salt and corn starch. Make sure they're thoroughly blended.
2. Combine the sweet almond oil and the essential oils. Add them to the dry ingredients and stir them in.
3. Add water or witch hazel to a spray bottle and use it to lightly mist the bath bomb mixture. Use

your hands to knead the liquid in until the mixture is slightly damp and is able to hold its form when you squeeze a ball of it in your hand.

4. Press the mixture into your bath bomb molds. Pack it as tightly as possible

5. Remove the bath bombs from the molds and place them in a cool, dry place for a day or two until they've had time to finish drying.

6. Store them in an airtight container in a cool, dry place.

Peace and Harmony

If you're an emotional wreck and your state of mind is feeling out of balance, this bath bomb might bring things back to center. I use one of these bath bombs whenever I'm feeling anxious or feel panic starting to set in, and it never fails to make me feel better.

Ingredients:

2 cups baking soda
1 cup citric acid
¼ cup Epsom salt
¼ cup corn starch
1 tablespoon sweet almond oil
5 drops geranium essential oil
5 drops lavender essential oil
5 drops sandalwood essential oil
Water or witch hazel

Directions:

1. Combine the baking soda, citric acid, Epsom salt and corn starch. Make sure they're thoroughly blended.
2. Add the essential oils to the sweet almond oil and stir them in.
3. Add water or witch hazel to a spray bottle and use it to lightly mist the bath bomb mixture. Use your hands to knead the liquid in until the

mixture is slightly damp and is able to hold its form when you squeeze a ball of it in your hand.

4. Press the mixture into your bath bomb molds. Pack the molds as tightly as possible

5. Remove the bath bombs from the molds and place them in a cool, dry place for a day or two until they've had time to finish drying.

6. Store them in an airtight container in a cool, dry place.

A Walk Through the Forest

If you're trying to convince your husband or significant other to try bath bombs, this might be a good one to toss in the tub. The warm, earthy fragrance of cedarwood is masculine enough to where it might just entice him to hop in.

Try blending other oils like citrus oils into this recipe to create interesting fragrance blends.

Ingredients:

2 cups baking soda
1 cup citric acid
¼ cup Epsom salt
¼ cup corn starch
1 tablespoon sweet almond oil
10 drops of cedarwood atlas oil
Water or witch hazel

Directions:

1. Combine the baking soda, citric acid, Epsom salt and corn starch. Make sure they're thoroughly blended.
2. Combine the cedarwood atlas oil and sweet almond oil and stir them together. Stir the wet ingredients and dry ingredients together.
3. Add water or witch hazel to a spray bottle and use it to lightly mist the bath bomb mixture. Use your hands to knead the liquid in until the

mixture is slightly damp and is able to hold its form when you squeeze a ball of it in your hand.

4. Press the mixture into your bath bomb molds. Pack the molds as tightly as possible

5. Remove the bath bombs from the molds and place them in a cool, dry place for a day or two until they've had time to finish drying.

6. Store them in an airtight container in a cool, dry place.

Piña Colada

All that's missing from this bath bomb is a little drink with the umbrella in it. I'll leave it up to you whether you want to have an adult beverage or two in hand while sitting in the tub with this bath bomb going, but it definitely evokes feelings of sitting in a tropical paradise.

This bath bomb calls for piña colada fragrance oil instead of essential oils because I've yet to find an essential oil blend that gets the smell right. Look for a plant-based blend for best results.

I like to color this bath bomb yellow using a natural yellow clay and then I press it into a pineapple-shaped candy mold I found online.

Ingredients:

2 cups baking soda
1 cup citric acid
¼ cup Epsom salt
¼ cup corn starch
1 tablespoon extra-virgin coconut oil
10 to 20 drops of piña colada fragrance oil
Water or witch hazel

Directions:

1. Combine the baking soda, citric acid, Epsom salt and corn starch. Make sure they're thoroughly blended.

2. Gently melt the coconut oil if it's solid. Add the fragrance oil to the coconut oil and stir it in.
3. Add water or witch hazel to a spray bottle and use it to lightly mist the bath bomb mixture. Use your hands to knead the liquid in until the mixture is slightly damp and is able to hold its form when you squeeze a ball of it in your hand.
4. Press the mixture into your bath bomb molds. Pack the molds as tightly as possible
5. Remove the bath bombs from the molds and place them in a cool, dry place for a day or two until they've had time to finish drying.
6. Store them in an airtight container in a cool, dry place.

Tea Time

This bath bomb won't have much smell to it unless you add some essential oils to the mix. What it does feature is green tea and some crumbled tea leaves, which will add polyphenols to the bath water. Polyphenols protect cells against free radical damage and may improve antioxidant capabilities. Green tea can also help prevent sun damage, but shouldn't be used in lieu of sunscreen.

The dried tea leaves can make a bit of a mess in the tub, so if you want to avoid getting them everywhere, place the bath bomb into a fine mesh baggy before tossing it in the tub.

Ingredients:

2 cups baking soda
1 cup citric acid
¼ cup Epsom salt
¼ cup corn starch
3 tablespoons strong green tea
1 tablespoon crumbled dried green tea leaves
Water or witch hazel

Directions:

1. Combine the baking soda, citric acid, Epsom salt and corn starch. Make sure they're thoroughly blended.
2. Brew the green tea much stronger than you would if you were planning on drinking it. Add

the green tea to the dry ingredients and stir it in.
You'll only be able to add a little bit at a time or
you'll set off the baking soda and citric acid.

3. Add the crumbled tea leaves to the mixture and
   stir them in.
4. Add water or witch hazel to a spray bottle and
   use it to lightly mist the bath bomb mixture. Use
   your hands to knead the liquid in until the
   mixture is slightly damp and is able to hold its
   form when you squeeze a ball of it in your hand.
5. Press the mixture into your bath bomb molds.
   Pack the molds as tightly as possible
6. Remove the bath bombs from the molds and
   place them in a cool, dry place for a day or two
   until they've had time to finish drying.
7. Store them in an airtight container in a cool, dry
   place.

59781032R00035

Made in the USA
San Bernardino, CA
07 December 2017